Sleep Medicine: Now!

"A monograph covering the basics of

the evolution of sleep medicine"

By:

Krystle Minkoff

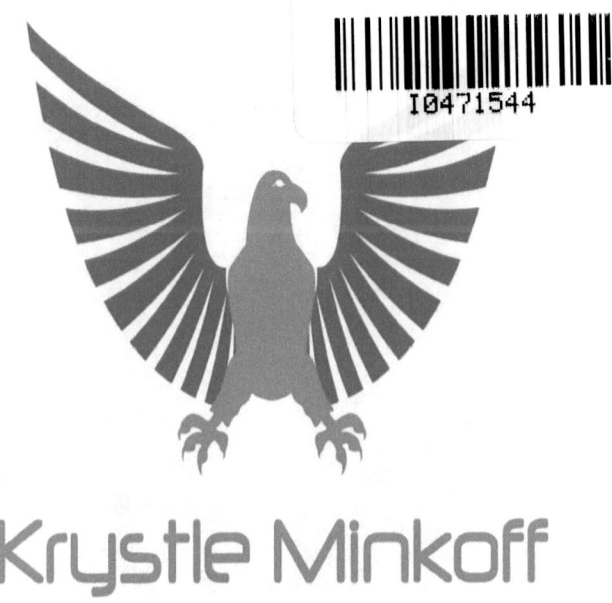

Krystle Minkoff

Sleep Medicine: Now!

Sleep Medicine: Now!

This book is dedicated to sleep professionals of all backgrounds and hopes to serve the purpose of enlightenment and continuing medical education in this ever evolving field of sleep.

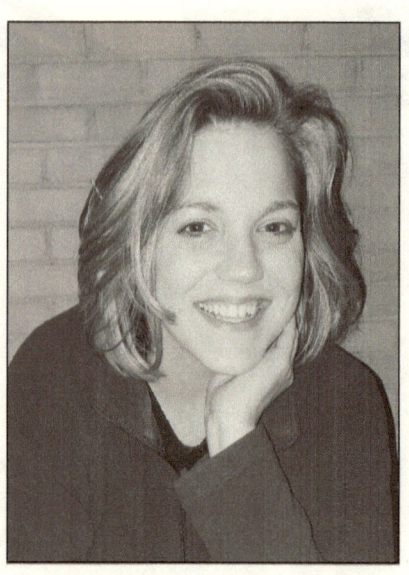

Table of Contents

I.   CPAP vs. APAP

II. HST vs. PSG

III. Sleep: A Progressive Field

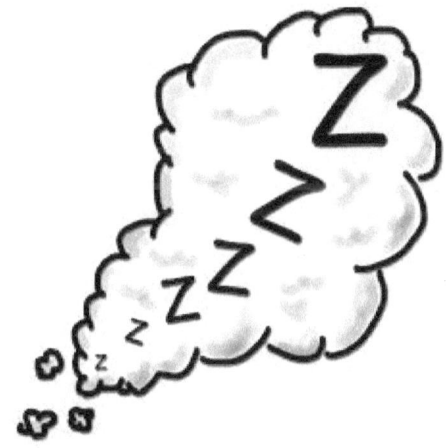

CPAP vs. APAP

Abstract:

I. Introduction

The purpose of this article is to examine the differences between CPAP vs. APAP & the efficacy of differences in the treatment forms.

II. Methods

The editorial is composed from specific professional knowledge as it pertains to sleep medicine from an industry expert who carries 15 years of experience within the field. Therefore, this is an original piece in its entirety with no references to cite.

III. Discussion

The reader will be able to effectively communicate on the efficacy differences between CPAP & APAP as it pertains to outcomes, cost, testing measures, and

convenience.

CPAP vs APAP

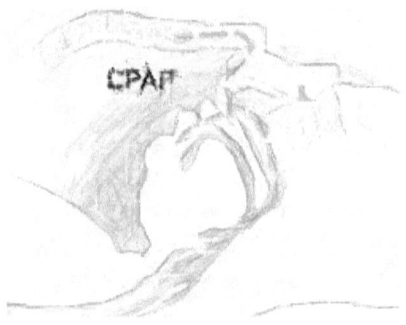

CPAP opening the airway

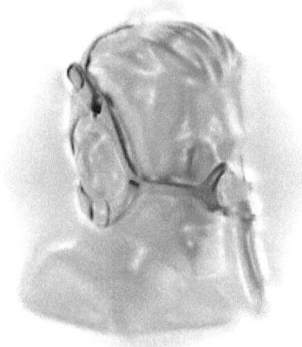

A standard nasal pillows CPAP mask

As we delve into the specifics of PAP (positive airway pressure) treatments for OSAS, this article begs to relay the differences in efficacy of CPAP (continuous positive airway pressure) vs. APAP (automatic positive airway pressure).

We shall begin with a subtle review of sleep apnea. Sleep apnea is a condition where there is an obstruction to the flow of air (and oxygen) during sleep, resulting in poor night time sleep and consequent daytime sleepiness. Should sleep apnea remain uncontrolled, this may contribute to elevated blood pressure, and an increased risk of stroke and heart attack.

The treatment of choice for OSAS has primarily and historically been CPAP (continuous positive airway pressure). CPAP is the only 100% effective therapy in treating OSAS. We shall attempt to make comparisons to investigate the differences, pros & cons, and efficacy of treatment between CPAP vs. APAP.

CPAP devices are titrated to a single set pressure setting by a sleep specialist. The titration study is conducted after a traditional in-lab polysomnogram test and is intended to solicit the exact pressure setting needed to alleviate or eliminate the majority, if not all apnea events during the night.

Contrary to the delivery of a single set pressure, APAP machines have a complex algorithm that detects on a breath-by-breath basis what pressure the patient needs at that and adjust accordingly. In essence, the APAP device finds the ideal pressure for any given moment.

It could be argued that one of the "cons" of CPAP that the single pressure may be cumbersome to tolerate (especially at higher settings), and doesn't adjust to varying pressure needs throughout the night. More and more frequently APAP devices are being prescribed in lieu of CPAP devices because of their versatility and ability to adapt to patient needs over the course of the night.

While APAP machines are costlier, APAPs can also be set to a single pressure. If for some reason APAP therapy isn't working well for the patient, they wouldn't need to get a different machine. APAPs can be set to a straight CPAP mode. CPAP devices on the other hand are unable to be adjusted to have multiple pressure settings.

APAP machines may be better intended for those that toss and turn during the night. Due to gravity, when you are supine you will have the most number of respiratory events in this position vs. being lateral or prone. This being said, the APAP automatically adjusts the pressure upward when severe events are detected and lower accordingly after positional and respiratory changes are apparent.

CPAP machines do not allow for physical changes, such as weight loss. It is recommended that if you have a 10% increase or decrease in body weight that the subject should undergo another evaluation to determine if a pressure increase or decrease is warranted. APAP devices can help eliminate the need for expensive in-lab sleep tests.

When you have a Home Sleep Test (HST) you will most likely be prescribed an APAP device. This is because HSTs can't determine which stages of sleep you are in. As previously discussed, CPAP devices are calibrated for breathing needs when you're at your worst (during REM sleep). HSTs score a period of your breathing needs through the course of the night to determine which range you need. With APAP, the range can later be fine-tuned with remote monitoring.

APAP therapy is swiftly becoming the go-to machine for treating OSAS as the technology becomes better developed. However, there are some instances where CPAP device may be the better choice:

- APAP manufacturers use a different algorithm to determine the patient's pressure ranges. This may make it difficult for some doctors to determine the best machine for their patients.

- The changes in pressure settings can ultimately be slow to react to the ideal pressure needs.

- APAP machines are not ideal for patients who, once starting treatment are discovered to have central sleep apnea; in which case an ASV or BiPAP machine may be the better suited.

- For patients with certain comorbidities, APAP machines are not recommended. These would include conditions such as chronic heart failure or obesity hypoventilation syndrome.

- While APAPs fluctuate between a high and low pressure setting, these settings need to be fine-tuned over time.

HST vs. PSG

Abstract:

I. Introduction

The purpose of this article is to examine the differences between HST (Home Sleep Testing) vs. PSG (Polysomnogram

II. CME (Continuing Medical Education)

This article intends to serve the purpose of providing a summarized perspective on the differences between home sleep testing and in center polysomnograms.

III. Discussion

The reader will be able to effectively communicate on the efficacy differences between HST & PSGs as it pertains to outcomes, cost, testing measures, and convenience.

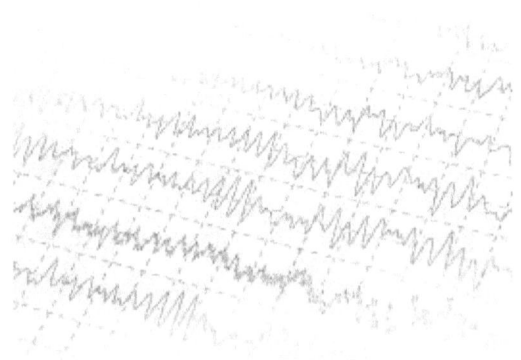

EEG (Electroencephalogram)

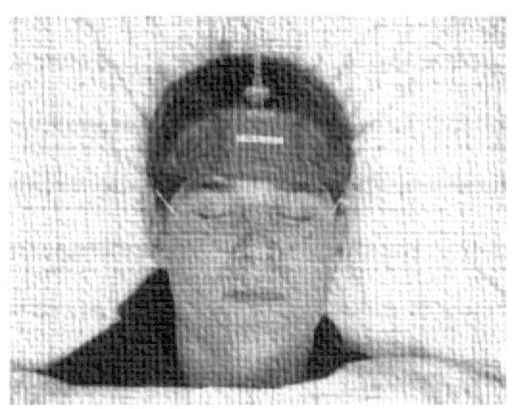

Standard HST

(Home Sleep Testing) device

Steadily becoming a popular option, HST is being performed with increasing prevalence due to its cost effectiveness and its ability to be done inside the home. This article attempts to draw comparisons to the significant differences between home sleep testing and in center testing better aka, HST vs. PSG.

As of today, current HST methods are not as comprehensive as a PSG. Polysomnograms can accurately monitor sleep stages, blood oxygen levels, respiratory effort and airflow, limb movements, muscle activity, heart rate and body position. HSTs are unable to measure the Respiratory Disturbance Index (RDI). This can result in subtler breathing irregularities being missed.

In addition to this, if the patient's results are determined to be borderline, only an in center test can rule out OSAS. This translates to the patient having to complete two procedures vs. one. In a sleep center, professionals monitoring the patient ensure the correct placement of equipment, ongoing integrity of the recording, and the correct measurement of important variables. However, due to their convenience for some patients, HST methods do have their competitive advantages over PSGs.

The question we should ask ourselves is, under what conditions are the use of HST vs. PSG appropriate? Currently, standards of practice indicate that PSGs are recommended to a patient if they suffer from comorbidities or another suspected sleep disorder, such as narcolepsy, insomnia, periodic limb movement disorder or a less known variant of sleep apnea called upper airway resistance syndrome (UARS).

As we continue to navigate the ever increasing use of HSTs, it is paramount to note the importance of being evaluated by an AASM accredited center with a board certified sleep physician. Adherence to a facility that maintains the gold standards of accreditation, by which stringent criteria are conceived and met can one be confident that their testing, results, and treatment outcomes are being met with the upmost quality of patient care.

Sleep: A Progressive Field

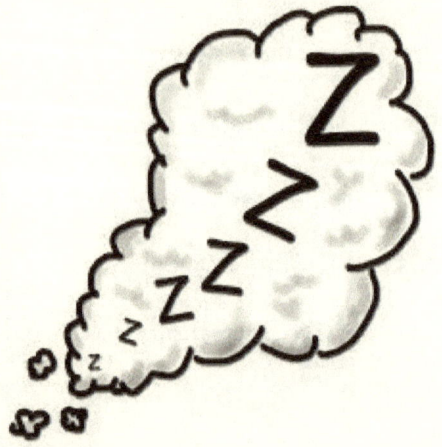

Sleep medicine has been a rapidly progressing field. It has seen unprecedented growth in the last 2 decades. It's estimated that throughout the United States in 1,292 sleep clinics, at least 1.17 million people were examined during 2001. These numbers have likely doubled since then, and other countries have seen a similar growth in the field of sleep medicine. The heightened awareness of sleep disorders as the field has become more widely known and healthcare more readily available has no doubt contributed to this dramatic increase in sleep clinics and the number of polysomnographic recordings.

Examinations to diagnose breathing disorders in sleep are carried out much the same way as they were done 20 or 30 years ago by sleep specialists. The methodology and encompassing aspects of diagnosis, treatment, and lab testing procedures have impressively advanced in ways that affect patients', outcomes, and insurance carriers. For one: Electrophysiological recordings have moved from analog to digital, and data are no longer stored on novel amounts of recording paper but on compact, miniature, digital storage media. This makes scoring of a digital polysomnographic record more precise and efficient.

As a result of the advances in sleep medicine, technology, and awareness insurance carriers have become more involved in defining the treatment and diagnosis parameters that affect the flow of testing and treatment. For years, the gold standard in sleep medicine included completing a comprehensive in-lab sleep study fully attended by a technician. Modern determinations geared toward more cost effective and speedier result outcomes have caused most initial testing to shift from the center based testing to in-home testing with portable devices.

These devices while not as comprehensive as an in center test can screen patients for significant apnea easily eliminating the need for a costly $2,000 procedure requiring the services of a technician and a setting with which to test overnight.

However, considerations have been made for patients with co-morbidities or who have a borderline result on the portable test. For these patients only an in-center sleep test attended by a registered technician and interpreted by a doctor whom is board certified in sleep medicine can rule out or positively diagnosis the sleep condition.

Treatment of apnea has now largely been automated with CPAP machines that use smart technology to detect patterns and algorithms in the patients' breathing and adjust the pressures to accommodate the patient's level of apnea through the night; seemingly eliminating the need for a fixed pressure such as CPAP (Continuous Positive Airway Pressure). Now, the treatment of choice is APAP (Auto Positive Airway Pressure). In large part, insurance carriers are now requiring physicians to prescribe APAP for straightforward cases of apnea vs. having a CPAP test in the facility to determine a fixed setting.

This is not only considered to be more efficient in streamlining the diagnosis to treatment ratio, but is considerably more cost effective. As awareness, access to healthcare and advances continue to progress in healthcare it is expected that there will continue to be an ever growing need for knowledgeable people to test, diagnosis, and liaison the care of patients with sleep disorders.

However, the atmosphere roles, technology, and methodology will continue to change.

Meet The Author

Krystle Minkoff

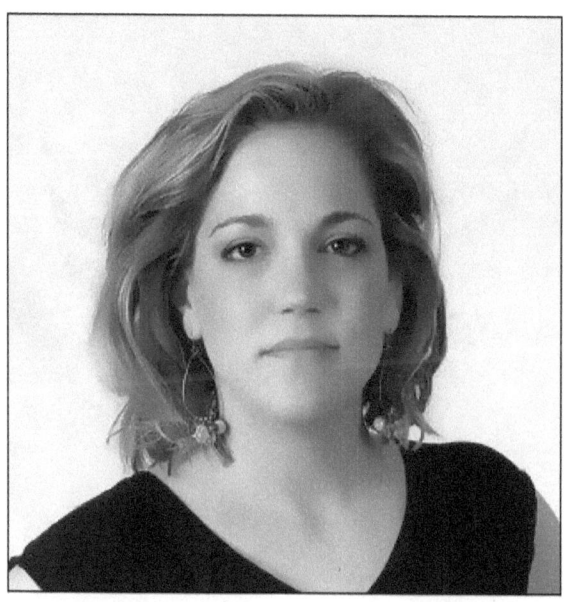

Krystle was born and raised in DFW, Texas. In a short period, her success as an audio-book narrator has demanded extensive commitments. She also stays busy as an actress, poet, and published author.

"Change is the law of life and those who look only to the past or present are certain to miss the future".

JFK-

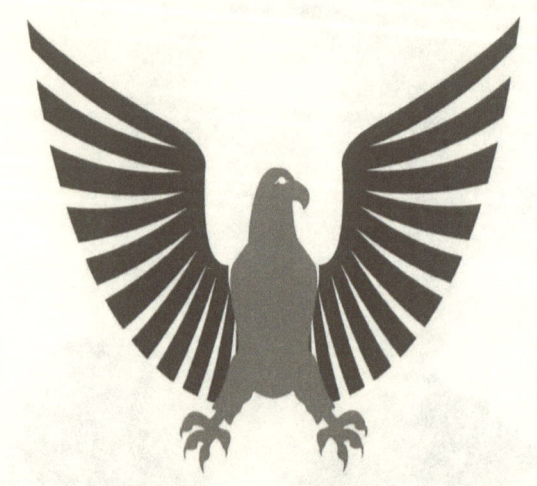

Krystle Minkoff

www.ingramcontent.com/pod-product-compliance
Lightning Source LLC
Chambersburg PA
CBHW030704190526
45164CB00004B/458

* 9 7 8 1 5 4 6 4 1 9 3 8 9 *